Behind Every Pill, There is a Story

By

Renee Lovett

Published by Lightning Source, a subsidiary of
Ingram Press Publishers

Available through Ingram Press, and available for
order through Ingram Press Catalogues

ISBN 978-1-62747-022-3 (paperback)

ISBN 978-1-62747-023-0 (ebook)

Printed in the United States of America

Visit my website @ PayingforPrescriptions.com

Acknowledgements

Thanks to my husband, Bill, for always
being there to bait my hook.
Thanks to my daughter, Lena, for always fixing my hair.
Thanks to my son, Dalton, for always making me laugh.
Also, thanks to Dr. Winer and Dr. Orbach from Winer
Wellness Center and Jean Liu, acupuncturist, for healing
me and my family, to Sam-I-Am for the inspiration to
write a book, to Mary Gardner, author and English
Professor, for believing in me, to Larry, Paulette, Allen
and Ashley for the opportunity to work with you, to Tom
Bird, Ramajon (finally got Word downloaded), Sherri
and Natalie for, without you guys, this would just be a
dream, to my sister, Lisa, for helping me to remember
childhood memories, and to my mom and dad for putting
up with my s*** all these years.
In loving memory of my Grandpap, Michael Kucinic,
because in Heaven there is no beer so that is
why we are drinking here!

Epigraph:

". . . each man's job is not just his job alone, but a part of the greater job whose horizons we at present can only dimly imagine. . ."

—Charles Drew

Chapter 1

"I will help you put on your ice skates for you," Bob would tell me every time my friends and I would go ice-skating.

Bob really liked me. He would diligently lace up my skates for me every Friday night. Then, Bob would follow me and my friends around the ice-skating rink, trying to get me to hold his hand and skate with him. One Friday night, I got tired of Bob asking me to hold his hand so I agreed to his hand-holding proposition. We were now considered boyfriend and girlfriend. Bob really wasn't my type, but he was my boyfriend now so I tried my best to like him. Bob was very smart, one of the smartest boys in our school. He was very tall and husky and had a very deep voice just like his dad, who was the local pharmacist when I was young.

After visiting the doctors, my mom would drive to a little store on the main street in the neighboring town. It was a small, red brick building that you had to climb several cement steps to get to. Once you opened the big glass doors, you were standing there looking at a very large guy who stood on a platform looking down at you. Yes, this was Bob's dad. He spoke in a very deep voice to my mom about pills. He then would say something funny to my sister, Lisa, and I, and then he would laugh a very deep, belly-sounding Santa Claus laugh. Lisa and I would meander across the shelves below the platform and look at all of the colorful candy and candy bars available. We would ask my mom if she could buy us some candy, and then Bob's dad would hand my mom the prescription and we would walk out through the glass doors, down the cement steps, and back into our car.

I was surprised one day when I went to Bob's house. He lived in a regular house like I did. It was actually fairly small for a family of five. Bob and his brother had to share a bedroom. When I went to the bathroom at Bob's, there was a glass bowl filled with tiny bars of soap. You know how you get to the end of a bar of soap and it becomes useless trying to hold it in your hand. Then, it slips out of your hand and falls in the shower. Well, apparently, Bob and his dad weren't the only smart ones in the family because Bob's mom told me that she would wait till the soap bowl was filled and then she would melt all of the little bars of soap and mold them into big bars.

It's nice that Bob's mom was thrifty with soap because life is full of uncertainties. You don't know from one day to the next whether you will have a job, whether you will be able to make your house payment, whether your investments will be up or down or whether you will be able to pay for your prescriptions. But what you can do is try to have a deep understanding of yourself and others. Look past yours and others' everyday routines. Take the time to get to know someone new. If you get to know a person, even if the two of you are so different from each other, you will, hopefully, find at least one thing that the two of you Have in common, whether it be an opinion, a common hobby, a favorite food, etc.

Really, how different can we possibly be? There are only so many religions, colors, hobbies, careers, and so on out there that we have to be alike in some manner. Take, for instance, prescription drugs. The drugs America spent the most money on in 2010 are:

1. Lipitor
2. Nexium
3. Plavix
4. Advair Diskus
5. Abilify
6. Seroquel
7. Singulair
8. Crestor
9. Actos
10. Epogen (DeNoon, 1)

Already, you may have a lot in common with another person because you may take the same drug or class of drugs as they do. And, also, by reading this list (if you take one of these above drugs or their generic counterparts), you probably feel a lot better knowing you're one of many people who take a medication such as these.

You are not the only one paying for them also. Taking your hard-earned cash out of your pocket each month to purchase your prescriptions. We would all like to have that extra money we spend on drugs to spend it on something we would enjoy, like going to the movies, eating out, or shopping for something we like. In 2010, Americans spent $307 billion on medications (DeNoon, 1). That's a lot of movies, popcorn, dinners, lunches, golf clubs, vacations, shoes, etc. we could have bought were it not for our medications.

Let's sit back, think, and ask ourselves this question: How have I accumulated my medications throughout my years of living? In most cases, you were not on ten pills the day after birth like you may be on now.

We all live life day to day. Life is busy. We are all working toward goals. Maybe we start out with the hopes of starting a family. We all want the best for our children. Our children take us through trials and tribulations. Sometimes we win our battles. Sometimes we lose our battles. In between career and family, we occasionally fall sick or experience pain and we need to see a doctor or visit a hospital. We accumulate medicine we must take through the years. Through everyday life, no fault of our own.

Now, we are faced with paying for these accumulated medicines.

Let's just pick an age, any age, let's pick, for the heck of it, age sixty-five. It's a generation of baby boomers. Now, like most older adults, each probably remembers vaguely being a child with maybe little or no health care coverage. However, not too many people visited doctors and hospitals back then. Perhaps when the now older adults reached their twenties, each maybe got a job with some union health benefits. What was the premium a month for their health care coverage? In a lot of cases: nothing. The health benefits were paid for by the unions. Sure, you paid your union dues but you didn't have that health care premium automatically deducted from your paycheck every month. However, some of these same older adult workers were not union workers, in which case, these families had no health care coverage whatsoever. When this group of "uninsured Americans" went to the doctor or a hospital, each was required to either pay the bill in full or make payments. Let's take, for example, my parents: it took them two years each to pay the cost of having my sister and I delivered at the hospital, for a total of four years.

How about prescription drugs back then? Ask some of these older adults and they won't remember. And the reason they can't remember isn't because they are getting older. It's that there weren't a lot of drugs prescribed forty-some years ago.

Ok. So we, as Americans, buy one-third of the world's drugs (Sager). Wouldn't you think we deserve a little discount then? After all, we go to big discount stores where we shop in bulk and get a little price break. If we buy a case of ketchup, we usually pay less per bottle than we do if we buy an individual bottle of ketchup. So it should be the same for prescription drugs, right?

Wrong. Let's take in the early 1990s for example: we, as Americans, paid thirty-two percent more for our drugs than the Canadians (Sager). They live right above us. So let's say we would have paid what the Canadians paid in the 1990s for the same drugs. How much money

would Americans have saved? Well, the answer is
$16.2 billion (Sager). Yes, that's billion. It's not a typo.

Did you realize we are "subsidizing" other nations'
drug costs? Why do we have to pay all this extra
money? Do Americans not like to have extra money in
their wallets to spend it on things we most enjoy?

Why isn't our government standing up against drug
companies to fix this disproportionate situation?

Getting back to our older adults who raised their
families on little health care costs and tried their best to
save for retirement, the golden years. Going by what
they were spending back then and adjusting for
inflation, some may have saved quite wisely. But what
they didn't foresee (and who could have?) was the costs
of prescriptions rising about three times as fast as
overall health costs (Sager). Multiply that number by
the number of prescription drugs taken by any one
individual.

It's as if you work all your life to pay for your
prescriptions. Let's take a look at Rose Ann. Rose Ann
is taking matters into her own hands. Her husband's
health has declined and Rose Ann is faced with a lot of
bills. After being retired for seven years, she went to
work for her neighbor. Rose Ann's neighbor is a single
dad trying to raise three boys. With the rising costs of
day care, Rose Ann's neighbor asked her if she knew
anybody interested in babysitting. And, with her
husband's health and their debts building, Rose Ann
decided to do it herself. So Monday through Friday
during the summer, she walks to her neighbor's house
and tries to keep track of three boys. In the past, Rose

Ann could talk your ear off. I would call her on the telephone and she would just talk and talk. An hour would go by and Rose Ann was still talking. I talked to her the other day and she didn't have much to say. She sounded exhausted. I said, "Rose Ann, how is your babysitting job going?"

And Rose Ann said, "I'm tired. Sometimes the boys run out of the house and I can't find them for hours. But the extra money helps pay for our health care costs and prescriptions."

Let's now stay on the same page here (not literally but mentally). Let's take a look at the up close and personal story of my parents and grandparents, so we can realize how alike and different we all are. How all of us, at one point in time or another, were young and unknowing. Unknowing of what was ahead of us. Unknowing of what could happen—either good or bad. Unknowing of what we were going to become. Unknowing of what pill we will need to take. We all have childhood memories whether it be looking for four-leaf clovers or helping mom get ready for a picnic, grilling outside, getting ready to go for a summer car ride, or going to our grandparents' house.

Chapter 2

G etting sick and staying home from school when I was young was awesome. I'd nap on the couch. The couch was made of felt-like dark blue raised designs on this rough, bluish fabric. Lying there all day on the couch, I would listen to Mom with her Dr. Scholls wooden clogs shoes on in the kitchen, washing dishes, preparing meals, doing laundry. The washing machine and dryer were downstairs in the basement and the steps going down were not carpeted. Clunk, clunk, clunk, down the steps, clunk, clunk, clunk, back up the steps. Mom did more laundry than anyone I've ever known, always in her cloggy shoes. I don't know why she thought the shoes were remotely comfortable. The bottoms were made of wood and the top had a gold metal buckle across the toes. I think she changed colors of the straps maybe once a year. Some years the strap was red, some years it was blue, sometimes, I think it was mostly red. Maybe she always had the same pair 'cause I had to have the latest and greatest Jordache jeans. And her toenails were always painted up perfectly. Her second toe on one foot was longer than her big toe. But her feet always looked spectacular.

She would make me dippy eggs and toast when I was sick. The eggs were never broken and the toast always perfect: very soft, not hard, and crusty, butter slathered on with cinnamon and sugar. I can still smell the cinnamon mixed with the smell of the eggs. She would bring it to me on a tray in the living room on the felt-raised blue couch that sat on the red rug. The rug had little raised balls on it. Strange material for a rug.

My grandpa lived on the other side of our house. It was a duplex. He was old-fashioned, but that didn't bother me, though. I didn't know what old-fashioned meant at that time. Grandpa would give us money every time the ice-cream man would come. Ding, ding, dong. The music played the "It's a Small World" song.

"It's a world of laughter. A world of tears. It's a world of hopes. And a world of fears. There's so much that we share. That it's time we're aware." Ding, ding, dong. "It's a small world after all."

Grandpa gave us grape bubble gum every day, and red pop, Cherokee Red soda in a glass bottle. We would give him back the glass bottles and my dad would drive Grandpa to town for the bottles to be cleaned and refilled (kind of like the old glass milk bottles).

Grandma Lena passed on so Grandpa thought my mom should cook for him. Like breakfast, lunch, and dinner, and, like, at specific times, like, very specific times. Dinner was at four o'clock. Not one minute after, not two minutes before, but four o'clock. That just didn't fly one day. I don't know why.

One day, my dad walked up the sidewalk after working hard all day and my mom said, "No more."

She's all flushed: red cheeks, her freckles aglow. Maybe it had to do with sometimes my grandpap would have happy hour, but it wasn't happy hour, it was happy hours. Then it would turn into happy days, and not the television show, either. And it wasn't rum and cokes, it was whiskey. And it wasn't just a shot of whiskey, it was bottles. I don't know. These are just things I heard through the years.

Grandpa was always just a barrel of fun in my eyes, though. He was always dressed to a "T" even though he only left the house once a week. He wore a dress shirt and suit jacket and dress slacks every day. When he'd leave town once a week to go to the bank, truck stop, and grocery store (after Mom stopped cooking for him), he'd put his dress hat on. He looked like a sharp-dressed man. He wore black dress shoes all shined up every day, whether he was in the house or outside. When Lisa, my sister, and I would play music, no matter what song it was, he'd tap dance with his shiny black shoes and sing "Rag Time Cowboy Joe." What we were playing was "Rhinestone Cowboy" by Glen Campbell. But after a few whiskeys, who cares what the words were?

Grandpa and Mom lived under the same roof for years, shared the same yard, but never spoke again. I had to go over to Grandpa's every day twice a day when I got older to give him his insulin shots.

Grandpa loved groundhogs. He gave them all the same name: "Bo-Bo."

When I turned sixteen, it was time to hit the road with Grandpa on his weekly excursion to the bank, to the truck stop, and to the grocery store. Stylish hat on his head, and now cane in his hand, off we'd go. It never failed; there was always a dead groundhog on the road.

"Poor Bo-Bo," Grandpa would say. "He went to town to buy a new pair of shoes and got hit by a car."

Back in the day, back before iPods, iPads, iPhones, and iThings, truck stops had little jukeboxes and there was one at each table. Every Saturday, like clockwork, Grandpa would give me some quarters and I'd play the jukebox while we sat and ate lunch together. And every Saturday, like clockwork, I would play the same song, "Old Time Rock and Roll" by Bob Seger:

"Just take those old records off the shelf. I'll sit and listen to 'em by myself. Today's music ain't got the same soul. I like that old time rock n roll."

I wouldn't play any other song. Two quarters, four songs, all four songs, "Old Time and Rock and Roll." Grandpa would ask me sometimes, "Hey, Nay, why don't you ever play anything else?"

"I don't know, Grandpa. I like this song," I would answer.

Amy, my childhood friend, lived two houses down. She wore short shorts with white around the edges and high white tube socks with stripes around the tops. Amy was bossy. She always told me what to do. And when I had another friend over, Amy would beat me up. She'd push me and punch me. But the next day, my friend would go home and Amy and I were the best of friends again. Amy was a cheerleader and would teach me cheers all day. Then, at the end of the cheer, we would have to end it in some elaborate stunt, which would mean she'd throw me in the air and I'd usually land flat on my face. Or she'd make me stand on her shoulders and then she'd get too tired and drop me. My head would bounce off the ground and I wouldn't be able to see straight for a couple of minutes or breathe for a few seconds. I think they call those concussions now. Maybe Amy was paying me back for having other friends over.

Amy and I. We danced a lot, too. When we weren't cheering, we were dancing. We would tape songs on a cassette, take our cassette player around the neighborhood, knock on peoples' doors, and ask if we could put on a dance recital for them. I can still remember "Another Brick in the Wall" by Pink Floyd playing on the cassette recorder. "All in all it's just another brick in the wall," and we would take our long, skinny legs with our short shorts and tube socks, and push off the side of the house (because it was made of bricks). We thought we were so cool doing that.

My mom took us to dance class at May-Lee's Dance Studio. May Lee didn't look like a dance instructor. But she taught us how to dance May Lee style. I can still remember, when you spin around fast, you have to pick one thing to focus on and every time you turn, you look at that same thing again, spin, again, spin, again, spin, again. Try it sometime. It really works.

Well, Amy decided that she and I were going to do a duet for the recital and she chose the song "The Stroke" by Billy Squier. We were in little neon green outfits that had sequins all over the tops. Two piece. And neon green arm bands that came up to our elbows. Amy wore lots and lots of makeup that day. Her lips were as red as a clown's nose. We were on stage dancing, she and I. Just wondering out loud here (WOL), what our parents were thinking. Maybe they just shrugged their shoulders and said, "That's the song Amy wanted to dance to, I guess." Maybe they had happy hour before the recital. Or perhaps they popped a Xanax.

Speaking of Xanax, Mom is no traveler of the seven seas. She prefers anything within a, let's say, twenty-mile radius of home. Dad tries to get her to go places but she adamantly refuses. Although one time, out of the clear blue skies, Mom announced she was taking us to California. For three weeks to boot. Her sister lives in California and we were going. I don't know if she was having a mid-life crisis. I'm just saying, you know. But, off we went.

So, every day, in California, my sister and I sat under my Aunt Betty and Uncle Ed's pool table with a deck of cards of the Dallas Cowboy Cheerleaders. Every day for hours, we'd go through the deck of pretty girls: there were black girls, there were redheads, there were blondes, many, many blondes. Texans must love their blonde cheerleaders. There were brunettes who were drop-dead gorgeous and there were brunettes who you wondered how they got in this deck of cards.

Lisa and I would take turns picking our cheerleading squad. Then we'd play with them for the rest of the day. Of course, they had cheerleading practice every day. And the pretty ones were always in the front and the not-so-pretty ones were in the back row. And when they made pyramids at the end of the cheer, the cute ones were always on the top (and they didn't fall off or get dropped on their heads).

We played cards until our older cousin, Kevin, who had very long legs, said, "I don't understand why you guys don't play a game with your cards."

So we'd sit down and play a card game called Spit with long-legged Kevin. And our Dallas Cowboy Cheerleader community would unravel and all the girls would be in one big pile, and they were just a number then.

Dad was by himself for three whole weeks. My dad never cooked anything in his whole life. We got back from California and all the tomatoes were off the plants. It wasn't even time for them to ripen and turn red yet. But they were gone. We thought Bo-Bo ate them all. But it turned out that Dad ate all the green tomatoes. For three weeks straight, my dad ate fried green tomatoes.

Chapter 3

Why do Americans take so many prescriptions? Some of us may take a drug because we may think something about our body isn't the same as it used to be when we were younger. Let's take, for instance, erectile dysfunction drugs. You may have thought you were normal before sitting down to watch your favorite television show, but after you see the commercial for a new drug and realized you have these particular symptoms, you may decide to call your doctor and get on this new drug. "Advertising drugs to the public often works by creating or exacerbating unhappiness or anxiety about symptoms or normal experiences. . ." (Carroll, 131). In addition to thinking we need a new drug for a new problem, some of us may think that our current drug isn't working as well as we think it should be. Perhaps a newer or more expensive drug on the market may do a better job. The ads we see on television are sometimes perceived as "medical breakthroughs." The pharmaceutical companies know that they are putting a lot of money into an ad for a new drug in hopes that a "medically gullible public" will ask for that particular drug at their next doctor's appointment (Gottfried, 20). In Critser's book,

Generation Rx: How Prescription Drugs Are Altering American Lives, Minds, and Bodies, he discusses how some older generic drugs worked fine for people for decades until money was spent on developing a newer drug designed to treat the exact same problem was developed (194-195). Also, Critser acknowledges the fact that the minimum ranges have changed throughout the years of people needing a specific drug for a specific problem, so that raises the amount of people actually needing the drug and it means a higher dosage for people already on a particular drug (193-194). One example of this is when researchers lowered the number for "bad" cholesterol to 100 when, previously, the level was 130 (Critser, 193). This meant that millions more people would be told by doctors that they need to lower their "bad" cholesterol, and consequently need to add another drug to their ever-growing pill case.

Chapter 4

L ike I said before, Mom doesn't like to leave town. One time we left town, though. We went five minutes up the road to a local hotel. It was a big to-do. Took my sister and me two days to pack everything. Barbie had to remember her swimming suit. She had to have matching high heels, sunglasses, outfits to lounge around the pool in, outfits for dinner that evening, outfits to run in . . . All of these outfits had to match a pair of shoes, you know, high heel shoes, of course. Our Barbie Dolls were finally prepared. We packed the car up, said good-bye to Dad, and off we went again on another adventure with Mom. We were there before you knew it. We unpacked all of our Barbie stuff all over the room. Now don't think for one minute there was nothing to do five minutes from home, 'cause there was. This hotel had a swimming pool. Barbie One and Barbie Two swam all day. I don't know what Dad ate for dinner that evening. Maybe fried green tomatoes. Maybe nothing. I got the feeling Mom didn't care for some reason that week.

See, Mom and Dad never fought. But maybe they did that week. Maybe Mom just needed an antidepressant.

Mom let Dad come on some vacations with us. About forty-five minutes from us is a zoo. Can you believe there are actually elephants, lions, giraffes, tigers, and bears in Pittsburgh? Ya, we couldn't, either. Our last vacation, we could see Interstate 70 and McDonalds from our hotel room. Well, this time, we could see a big highway and some buildings bigger than our hotel. Mom bought me and my sister matching Wonder Woman Underoos. Underoos were pajamas made to look like superheroes. That's all me and Lisa did was jump on the bed with our superhero pajamas on. We jumped for hours and then, the next day, we couldn't wait to leave the zoo to go back to the hotel to put our Wonder Woman Underoos on and jump on the beds. We jumped for hours until the alcohol from dinner wore off my parents and my dad said, "OK, enough jumping on the bed."

He probably wished he was home by himself, eating fried green tomatoes.

Chapter 5

The marketing of a drug through advertising to the public is just one factor in the consideration of why Americans end up on so many prescriptions. After getting through your mind that you need a drug, pharmaceutical companies also have to penetrate the minds of your doctor. In Marcia Angell's discussion about the unethical efforts of drug manufacturers to educate doctors, she quotes Jay S. Cohen of www.medicationsense.com: "Drug companies are subtle. They not only provide gifts and dinners and seminars, but also leave behind carefully selected studies that support the use of their drugs" (Carroll, 141). If your doctor is getting golf trips, gifts, vacations, etc. from a drug representative for prescribing a certain drug, the more apt your doctor is to recommend this drug to you. In Marcia Angell's book, *The Truth About the Drug Companies: How They Deceive Us and What To Do About It*, she discusses the role prescription-tracking companies have in getting information about what prescriptions doctors write, and then they report this information to the drug companies (129-130). Then, when the drug company sends its drug representative out to see a particular doctor, the drug sales representative knows if that doctor is using a competitor's drug (Angell, 130). After meeting with the doctor, after maybe a nice dinner and a game of golf, after maybe a generous supply of free samples, the doctor may be writing more prescriptions for this other company's drug, claiming to the patient that it may work better. Just to give you an idea of how widespread these practices are, "In 2005, pharmaceutical companies spent $7 billion on sales representative visits to physicians and provided $18 billion worth of free samples (Verbruggen, 76). Pharmaceutical companies wouldn't spend this kind of money on marketing if all of their marketing didn't pay off in the end. They have studied their investment and have found that if a doctor accepts pill samples, they will, in turn, write a prescription for that particular drug in the future. In fact, Carl Elliott, an author of many books on medicine and morality, states that "Drug reps may well have more influence on prescriptions than anyone in America other than doctors themselves . . ." (Carroll, 113).

Given the direct-to-consumer advertising and the doctors' financial willingness to prescribe a drug, it's no wonder why Americans are on so many prescription drugs.

Why do Americans pay more for their drugs than other countries? Let's take, for instance, five popular drugs in an article in *Consumer Reports* and compare the average retail price for a one month's supply. If you were a diabetic in Japan and take Actos for your condition, you will pay $21.48 for your one month's supply; however, if you are a diabetic in the United

States on the same medication, you will pay $86.13 for your one month's supply. The popular drug for cholesterol, Lipitor, in France is $19.53 for a one month's supply, but in America, it is $68.37 for a month's supply. How about Nexium for heartburn? An Australian will pay $22.23/month, but an American will pay $92.04/month. Continuing on here with the high cost of being from America with a health condition that requires taking a drug, in the case of asthma and the drug, Singulair, you will pay $83.40 per month, as opposed to being from the United Kingdom and paying $51.09 per month. Similarly, purchasing four pills of Fosamax for osteoporosis in Canada will cost $35.07, and purchasing the same in the United States is almost double, at $64.16 ("Six," 15).

Now, we all know that everybody doesn't pay full cost for their medicine, but the full cost of a drug will factor into the premiums we all pay for our health care costs. So, the higher the cost that an insurance company will have to pay for a particular medication, the higher the cost of the insurance will be and this will be passed on to the consumer. In the 1990s, prescription coverage was added to most insurance plans, whereas before, a lot of people just paid out of pocket for their medication, and as a result of this addition, it is now more costly for insurance companies to provide insurance coverage (Gottfried, 53). With the rising costs of prescription drugs and the rising utilization of them, drugs become a huge factor in the affordability of a health plan for employers to offer to their employees even though the drugs are only 20 percent of the total cost of an employer health care plan (Dietz, 38).

Still, with all of the health care coverage offered to many Americans, we are clearly using all of this coverage we are afforded rather frequently. As a study in 2009 of thirteen industrialized countries pointed out, the United States spent the most on health care at approximately $8,000 per person, as opposed to Japan spending the least on health care at approximately $2,878 per person ("US," 26). Employers are taking measures to contain these high costs by offering different incentives to employees and their insured family members for costs of their medicines. One of the most popular ways of saving on medications is choosing a generic drug over a brand-name drug (Dietz, 39). As Dennis Gottfried, M.D., a doctor for over twenty-five years, noted, "Even though these generic medications are often as effective as the costlier brand name medications, they are rarely promoted, because they are less profitable for the pharmaceutical companies" (54). Here again, advertising to the consumer about a new, better drug for the same problem may influence a person to want the new, better drug, which is always brand name, meaning a higher out-of-pocket cost for the consumer and a higher cost for the insurer insuring the person.

Chapter 6

M om did have a mom and dad she talked to. Her mom was even more homebound than her. Grandma Maisie didn't leave the farm. So, every Sunday afternoon in the summer, we would go sit on Grandma Maisie and Grandpa Jake's porch. It was an old-fashioned porch made of cement, and every time people would talk, their voices would echo. We sat and listened to the echoes of grown-ups talking. Grandpa Jake sat on the porch swing with his dog. His first dog, I can remember, was a pug dog. His name was "Puggy." Puggy sat on Grandpa's lap. Puggy didn't like Ralph. Ralph was the neighbor guy who sat in the corner of the porch. He didn't say much. He just sat there, and when somebody would laugh, Ralph would laugh. I don't think I ever heard Ralph talk. When we'd get to the top of the steps of the porch, my mom or dad would say, "Hi, Ralph." (Echo: Hi Ralph). "How are you doing?" (Echo: How are you doing?).

And Ralph would smile and shake his head. Ralph had long legs, too. But he's not related to us.

Grandpa Jake had really long legs, as matter of fact. Grandma Maisie only came up to the top of his legs. I remember seeing a picture of them the day they got married. I don't know how my Grandpa Jake found her. He probably walked around all the time, saying, "Maisie, Maisie, where are you?"

After Puggy died, Grandpa Jake got this annoying little wiener dog and it barked every time someone moved. And the barks were high pitched and they echoed on the porch. So nobody said much anymore. We just all sat there and all of us became Ralphs.

Summers at Grandma Maisie and Grandpa Jake's were actually cooler (temperature-wise) than visiting in the winter. Grandma Maisie's house was about ninety-five degrees in the winter. The coal furnace burned like crazy, which could be why we only visited once during winter, which was Christmas Eve. Either that or we just didn't have anything to say except "Merry Christmas."

There were a lot of people in that little farmhouse on Christmas Eve. We all wore short-sleeved shirts. My grandma sat on the heater until someone needed a can opened. That little, tiny woman opened cans with an old-fashioned can opener. The kind you turn with your hand to cut through the metal. We would all watch her in amazement. And every year, someone would buy her an electric can opener, but every year, she'd tell them, "Take it back. I have a can opener."

All the ladies would sit in the little kitchen and all the men would sit in the little living room and watch a tiny little television. One year, everybody pitched in and bought them a bigger television. The next year, someone asked Grandpa Jake, "How do you like the new television, Jake?"

He said, "The picture is too big. I wish I had my little one back."

There was always traffic in and out of the door going to the echoing porch. Not much conversation, either, besides, "It's so hot in here."

We all turned into Ralphs after ten minutes of being in the house. Except us kids, we didn't care. We were all shoved in the parlor, which was a tiny room with a couch, an old-fashioned organ with foot pedals, and my grandpa's puzzle-building table that wobbled. We had a blast in that room. For hours, we would take turns hiding under the hundred winter coats. I'm surprised no one ever passed out under those coats.

There was also a big curtain that had a big, white plastic end on the strings, which you used to open and close it. It looked like a razor, so we would emerge from the coats and say, "It's time to shave." Then, we'd act like we were shaving our beards.

Not much fuss or drama on Christmas Eve. When it was time to eat, Grandma would open a can of beets with her hand-held can opener and we'd all watch in amazement. Someone would shout, "Grandma is using the can opener," and all of us kids would stop shaving, emerge from the coats, and go watch.

This would startle a few of the men in the living room, who would then wake up and they would all say the same thing: "I got to go get some fresh air on the porch."

The ladies would all make their husbands a plate of food: lunchmeat and cheese sandwiches, a beet, and a pickle. They would then awaken the ones who weren't awake, hand them their plates, and ask them what they wanted to drink.

Until one year, my cousin, Tammy, decided to buck the system. Tammy, the feisty redhead that she is, decided she was <u>not</u> going to make her husband, Keith, a plate of food. She said, "He has two legs. He can come and get it himself."

This did not go over well with the other ladies in the kitchen.

There was much fuss.

"Tammy, just take Keith a sandwich," her mom said to her.

"No, I work just as much as him. He can come get his own sandwich."

Then, my mom said, "Oh, Tammy, I will make Keith a sandwich. What does he like on it?"

Being the bold redhead that she is, Tammy wouldn't tell my mom what Keith likes on his sandwich.

Meanwhile, in the living room with the little television, Keith was all of a sudden the center of attention. Everybody woke up for this show. For years, the women have served the men. What was going on here? Should Keith just sit there and take the humiliation and scrutiny of all the men with plates on their laps? Or should he stand up and be a manly man, and demand Tammy bring him a sandwich? What would you do if you were Keith? And if he does get up off his chair and head toward the kitchen, does he slump his shoulders over and surrender? Or does, he boldly get up, sigh in disbelief and adamantly prepare a sandwich for himself?

Keith didn't eat that Christmas Eve. He went home hungry. We all crawled in our little beds that Christmas Eve and thought about poor Keith. How is it that a man so nice, so quiet and innocent, had to go to bed hungry? What did he do to deserve this? He didn't do anything wrong. He was just born a man. The thing is, other men would have helped him out, but they were too scared. Too scared of what the other plate-bearing men would have thought. Sometimes, it's just best to call it a night and take an ambien.

Either my dad was so excited he wasn't married to Tammy or he had a really good day at work. I'm talking really good day at work. 'Cause there were some nights at dinner that we would sit down to eat and all my dad did the entire meal was laugh. He laughed so hard that we laughed at his laughing. We laughed so hard that I don't know how we ate dinner. There was no time to swallow food 'cause my dad would start laughing again. I could lean back on the two legs of my chair and my dad wouldn't even yell at me. He was too busy laughing to even notice. Maybe my dad took too many antidepressants that day or maybe he smoked some doobies after work.

Mom. She had different ways to blow off steam. Cigs. Ya, my mom was a cigarette smoker back in the day. She was a weird cigarette smoker, though. The only time she would smoke was when she was with her friend, Hoppy. You knew when the two of them got together, clear the room 'cause you weren't going to be able to breathe. When my mom smoked with Hoppy, she forgot she had kids. Hoppy had a son, Timmy.

Timmy was a redhead. Just saying. One day, Timmy and Lisa went outside to escape the smoke, and Timmy took a hold of Lisa's hair and pulled it as hard as he could. He pulled and pulled my sister's hair. And he wouldn't let go. My sister cried and cried, and Timmy wouldn't let go of her hair. He just stood there, smiling. I hope someday Timmy's wife makes Timmy make his own sandwich on Christmas Eve.

One day, Hoppy was at our house, and I walked through our kitchen and coughed and coughed, acting like I was dying. I fell to the floor, coughing, and laid there and said, "You're killing me. You're killing me with all of this cigarette smoke." Soon after, my mom quit.

Chapter 7

Whether it be generic or brand name, all of this medication is affecting our bodies. You would think that we are healthier now that we are taking all of these pills. In essence, when you think about how one of your appointments at the doctor's office may go, it may seem to follow some sort of pattern. You may go to the doctors for a certain symptom you are having; let's just say you have a headache that won't go away. Your doctor may order some tests to rule out any severe underlying problems. If none are found, he will probably prescribe a medicine to treat your headache symptoms. However, he is doing just that: he's treating the symptoms. Now, let it be known that he is not curing your problem. Without the medication, you will still have the initial problem, the headache, in this case. But we go about our daily lives now, with this new medication in hand, thinking that our doctor made us feel better and he did a great thing. We, as Americans, are so accustomed to this kind of treatment that it has become the acceptable norm. Our pills become like our cell phones. You feel lost without either one. They have become a part of us, a part of our bodies, a part of our daily routine.

One would now think that since we don't have a headache every day all day that we are better off than we were before. However, with our new headache medicine that we are taking, we now have a new problem that we have to deal with every day. Let's just say, for example purposes only, that we are constipated. Now, this warrants a second trip to our doctor's office, where we learn that constipation is just a side effect of our new headache medicine we are taking. So in order to combat this new problem, we need to take a new constipation medicine. Keep in mind that we still don't even know the real reason why we developed the headache in the first place.

With all of this medicine, Americans should be the healthiest people on the Earth. But "There are more than 106,000 deaths a year from serious adverse drug reactions" (Critser, 8). One major concern of many people in the field is liver damage. All the prescription drugs, all of the over-the-counter medications, and all of the supplements we take pass through our liver. FDA expert, John R. Senior, stated, ". . . drug-induced liver injury has become the leading cause for removal of approved drugs from the market, and for acute liver failure in patients evaluated at liver transplant centers in the United States" (Critser, 173).

One example of how acid reflux drugs affect our bodies is shown in Critser's book. These heartburn drugs are used by about 2.5 million Americans daily and they actually decrease stomach acid (Critser, 198). However, too little stomach acid can actually be unhealthy. "It can, for one, lead to a severe lack of properly digested minerals—minerals essential to the health of all key organs" (Critser, 199).

One may ask, then, why would a doctor prescribe a drug that may actually cause damage? Well, the answer to this question may be in the Flexner Report. This model shaped the way doctors treat their patients. They are all taught according to this modern-day model to treat the symptoms of a disease, not to cure the disease itself. The actual report does not say this directly. In 1906, Abraham Flexner, author of the infamous Flexner Report, which reformed medical education, inspected 155 medical schools in the United States and Canada, and found many to be unacceptable (Barr, 19-20).

Perhaps we need a current reevaluation of teaching our future medical doctors. Over 100 years ago, the Flexner Report was a needed improvement to our medical establishment. Learning and medical facilities were evaluated for their "acceptable quality" (Barr, 20). Minimum requirements were also being implemented by colleges, requiring four years of study, of which two were to be in a clinical setting (Barr, 18).

Today, the curriculum has obviously evolved and changed to require more education. However, it is still science-based learning. Our future doctors are still taught to treat the symptoms with medicine. If you ever wonder why a doctor writes a prescription for a pain medicine to treat your pain, it could be that is what he learned to do in medical school. The doctor wasn't taught to look at treating the actual cause of your pain. Some think that "we shift clinical education to a model that integrates disciplines and focuses on team-based learning 'so that health care professionals can come to a better understanding of their interdependence'" (Barr, 21). This sort of new and improved model of learning is much needed in today's environment, especially since there is a proliferation of psychologically-based medication. With the addition of social and behavioral sciences as part of the curriculum (Barr, 21), we can integrate this knowledge along with the clinical medical knowledge and work together in the best interest of the patient.

As health care evolves into a better practice for everyone, we can then envelop the benefits of medically-necessary medication. Dr. Marcia Angell states that drugs "should be prescribed carefully and only when necessary, and doctors' judgment about their prescription should be based on real research and education, not on the marketing that passes for it." (172). We can all hope that this happens in the future, as Americans are put on more and more drugs than ever before.

Chapter 8

Besides my grandma and grandpa's on Sundays, we didn't do much visiting except to our neighbor Ann's house. Ann was an older lady who liked to clean. Ann cleaned all day. From sunup to sundown, Ann cleaned. And when we went to visit her, she would tell my mom what she cleaned that day. The only time you saw Ann when we weren't visiting was when she would come out onto the porch to shake out her rugs. The only time we would visit Ann was when it would storm.

My mom hated storms, scared her to death. I think my mom knew when it was going to storm. Her cheeks would get all red and all her freckles would stand out on her face and arms, and her hair would get all messy from all the sweat. She'd prance back and forth with her Dr. Scholls on, clunk, clunk, clunk. She'd look out the porch window at the darkening sky. Clunk, clunk, clunk, she'd look out the kitchen window. "Let's go down Ann's," she'd say.

Ann would be all sweaty, too, 'cause she just spent all morning cleaning, so she'd say, "Let's just sit outside on the porch until the storm gets closer."

And when the storm would finally come, we'd go inside, and my sister and I would sit at Ann's kitchen table, eating all of her hard-tack sour balls.

There were some days that Ann wasn't home and we were stuck home with mom while it stormed. She would make us sit in the two feet by four feet hallway that went in between our side of the house and my grandpa's side of the house, with both the doors shut. It got as hot as my Grandma Maisie and Grandpa Jake's house in that hallway. Every time it would thunder, she'd put her arms up by her head and scrunch her head down. Then she'd peak up, half open her eyes, and wait for the lightning to flash. Finally, the storm would stop and she'd let us out of the hot hallway. We could breathe once again.

One day, Mom went back to work. She decided she was going to be a telemarketer. So she called people up on the phone and she asked if they wanted to buy something. And when they said no, like most did, she said, "OK," and hung up the phone.

My mom doesn't like bothering anyone about anything. She doesn't even like calling me on the phone now 'cause she thinks she might be interrupting me. When I call or visit her, she always says, "I was going to call you and tell you this or that, but I thought you were probably busy."

My poor sister, Lisa, took the chance and moved out of mom's twenty-mile radius of her house to a town twenty-one miles away. Mom never visits. Mom never calls, either. "Lisa's probably working," she says.

Mom always took care of us, so when she got the telemarketing job, we were all lost. She'd have specific instructions on how to heat up dinner and whose turn it was to do the dishes that night.

It was lonely without mom around. Dad was in the garage. Dad was always in the garage. It was Dad's escape from the world. Dad started on a car one day that was a chunk of rusted metal sitting on blocks in our yard. It was a frame of a car. I remember me, bossy Amy, and Lisa would duck underneath the blocks, get up under it, and stand up and pretend like were driving down the highway. My dad's friends would stop by and they'd all stand around with their arms crossed, their beer bellies pushed out, and just stare at the hunk of metal on blocks. One day, a kid from my class road by my house, and he asked me in school the next day what my dad was going to do with that frame sitting in our yard. I said my dad is going to make a car out of it. He laughed. I was so mad at him. Dave was his name. I was so mad at Dave. For years after that, I would pass Dave in the hallway and he'd ask, "Hey, Renee, how's your dad coming along on that car?" He'd always have a smirk on his face when he asked, "Does your dad have that car done yet?"

Well, I knew after that I'd never date a guy named Dave ever in my life.

My dad worked on that car every chance he got. If he wasn't at work or cutting grass, he was working on that car. I believed in my dad. Besides, I wanted to go to school one day and tell Dave, "My dad got that there car done and running, Dave."

Some days, I'd find Kitty, our outside cat, go sit on a chair in the garage, and watch Dad work on his car. Kitty would fall asleep on my lap and I'd ask my dad questions about what he's going to do next and, "Why are you doing that?" And, "Where does that piece go?"

Chapter 9

S ubsequently, we face the problem of paying for all of our accumulated prescriptions. A lot of people need help paying for their prescriptions. There are a lot of different ways Americans can get help. You may be able to receive help according to your income eligibility or through the drug manufacturer. There are sometimes federal or state help that you can apply for and organizations set up for specific diseases that will help with your medication costs. However, there is, unfortunately, not help for everyone all of the time.

It's sad when people have to make a choice over treatment with a recommended medication and not taking the recommended medication because of not being able to afford it. In many instances, people take their medication every other day to prolong its use. And some people cut their medications in half without being told to do so by their doctor.

Comparing the Medicare Part D prescription program with the VA drug plan, in 2006, Medicare started offering prescription drug coverage for Medicare eligibles ("Focus," 1). In 2009, there was about 72 percent of Medicare beneficiaries enrolled in these Medicare Part D plans ("Focus," 3). The VA drug program offers prescription drugs for eligible veterans. "Overall, the VA pays 52 percent below retail for its two dozen most commonly prescribed medications." The reason the VA can offer such a discount to their qualified veterans is that they negotiate prices with the drug companies. Medicare Part D programs do not negotiate prices with drug companies, as this practice is prohibited. Therefore, prices are much lower for those veterans eligible for VA drug benefits than those on a Medicare prescription plan. Drug companies love this, as this means more profits from Medicare beneficiaries (Gottfried, 76-77). Between the years 2006 and 2013, economist Dean Baker claims that if Medicare were able to directly offer their own Part D prescription plan and were allowed to negotiate their drug costs with pharmaceutical companies, then this would result in a savings of $600 billion (Carroll, 179-180).

The above example of how drug prices are negotiated is just a small example, but on a larger scale, there are other price negotiations going on. Individual countries also negotiate drug prices. Canada, Australia, Japan, France, and many other countries regulate prescription drug prices, but the United States does not (Angell, 219). Pharmaceutical companies do admit to the higher drug prices for Americans and claim that they need to compensate for the lower prices they charge other countries because Americans are able to foot the bill (Angell, 38).

We could go across the border to Canada and get our medications cheaper or we could get on the Internet and purchase our medications, but both concepts would probably not be a very good idea. "The U.S. Food and Drug Administration continues to warn the American public about the dangers of buying medications over the Internet. . ." ("Sacramento"). As for going to Canada to purchase your drugs, the United States is trying to protect Americans from counterfeit drugs so this practice is not recommended, either (Angell, 221).

With all of these regulations, recommendations, restrictions, and rules, we are still looking for some help with paying for our prescriptions. Look no further than Obamacare is what we are told anyway. Trying to figure out the new health care law will be difficult until we live with it for a while and then see if, really, what we were told is really helping us, or if we are actually paying more in taxes or surcharges or co-pays or coinsurances or whatever the government wants to call the extra that will be coming out of the pockets of Americans.

One aspect of the new health care program has to do with Medicare beneficiaries. With the Part D prescription coverage, there is currently what is referred to as the "donut hole," which is a term for the coverage gap between the initial coverage stage and the catastrophic stage. For people who fall into this stage, it means paying more most of the time for their prescriptions than they did when they were not in this stage of prescription coverage. With Obamacare, this "donut hole" will be slowly closed, and by the year 2020, there will be a 25 percent co-pay that Medicare beneficiaries will pay for generic and brand-name drugs (Altman, 328). This may sound good, but we may not know if this will actually save Medicare beneficiaries money until the program is actually in effect in 2020. Twenty-five percent of what price is what we should be asking. This amount could vary. It is usually cost effective to take a generic drug to save money, but not all persons are able to do this for various reasons. One reason being that a generic may not be available. Another reason is that a generic version of the drug may not work for that particular person as well as a brand-name drug works for them. The latest "trend," if we can call it a "trend," is for drug manufacturers to set the total cost of a generic drug at about the same price that the brand-name drug costs. We have seen this with the drug Lipitor and Atorvastatin. So, taking 25 percent of a higher amount is obviously not going to save you much money.

With these kinds of price differences between drugs, the actual cost of a drug has to be taken into consideration. "According to industry experts, it costs about $800 million to bring a new medication to market" (Gottfried, 54). What goes into this $800 million is questionable. We would all like to think that it is research. However, Dr. Angell points out that most research is done in laboratories at universities and within the government (22). Much of the expense is on advertising and marketing (Gottfried, 55). In one study done by the Department of Health and Human Services, doctors were paid for getting some of their patients in a new drug study $12,000 per patient (Angell, 30-31). A portion of this total cost of a drug being manufactured also goes to chief executive officers (Carroll, 160). As you can see, many factors go into the creation of a new drug, and after a patent expires and a generic drug is available, it is obviously less expensive. It usually takes seventeen to twenty years for a drug to go from brand name to generic. During the seventeen-to-twenty-year period that a drug is under patent protection is the time period when the pharmaceutical company that has the patent for the drug makes most of its money (Gottfried, 54). From a pharmaceutical company point of view, this is the time when they must market this new drug as the recent innovative miracle drug to sell more of this drug in this patent-protection period. Therefore, as previously discussed, the drug is advertised to the public as such. And, consequently, drug reps are handing out free samples to doctors and handing them literature that shows study after study (written by the drug companies) that this new, improved drug is worth prescribing to their patients. Dr. Gottfried, in his book, *Too Much Medicine: A Doctor's Prescription for Better and More Affordable Health Care*, gives this advice: "Medications within the same class of drugs are equivalent. Ask for generic substitutes" (54).

Taking a generic substitute is one way of lowering your overall drug costs. But if we take more than one drug, costs can add up quickly, especially if any of our drugs are brand name. Between the years 1992 and 2002, a study showed an increase in the number of drugs per person, taken from 7.3 to 11.6 (Dietz, 38). If doctors and pharmaceutical sales representatives were not profiting from prescriptions, possibly, prescription drug use would decrease instead of increase.

Chapter 10

One day, I decided: "Hey, I got to get the hell out of this small town. I'm going to fly across the country to Arizona and go to college."

My mom was sad. She knew there was no one who would take care of me there like she could take care of me here. "Who in heaven's name is going to cut the crust off your bread for you, Renee?"

So my mom threw a little party for me and invited my closest friends, Jen, Chelle, Mike, and Bill, who all looked at me and said, "Are you nuts?"

Well, Mom still supported me even though she knew I was lucky to find my way back and forth to the local mall and not get lost, let alone try to make it in a big city clear across the country.

So, like all women do: when all else fails, go shopping! Mom bought me the fluffiest towels ever. If there were ever an award for the most softest, fluffiest bath towels, these towels would have won.

Hope my dad did some overtime that week because we came home with a carload of fly-across-the-country stuff: cooking utensils, bowls, silverware, fluffy towels, bedsheets, pillows, corkboards, notebooks, and more fluffy towels. And, on the way home, Mom crossed the centerline and almost drove us off the turnpike. I thought to myself, *I'm not going to make it to Arizona to use my big, fluffy towels the way Mom's driving.* You see, her favorite man, besides my dad, Rod Stewart, came on the radio and sung "Forever Young."

Mom's hands tightened on the steering wheel and her knuckles got all pink. You couldn't even see her pretty, pink fingernails. They were tucked so tightly in her palms that she probably made herself bleed. Her eyes were aglow; tears were streaming down her face. Hell, she even made me cry and I didn't even know what we were crying about.

"May the good Lord be with you. Down every road you roam. And may sunshine and happiness. Surround you when you're far from home" (Rod Stewart).

Mom had stomach problems ever since. I'm sure I had nothing to do with that.

Bags packed. I was leaving town. Mom made Dad go with me, though. Lord knows I'd probably get on the wrong plane and end up in Alaska if he didn't. I didn't even know how to wash towels or clothes, but I was going to fly across the country with fluffy bath towels.

Dad and I flew to Arizona. He was sad. I could tell. Dad had to start taking blood pressure medication after he found out I was going away to college.

Or maybe the high blood pressure started after I totaled his car or maybe it was that stop sign that suddenly appeared at an intersection one day I was driving or maybe it was that mailbox that started moving one day and left that big scratch on the new car Dad just bought me. I don't know. Never will know.

All I know is that the day before my dad left Arizona, I was getting ready for bed in the hotel bathroom and I came out, and my dad had the porn channel on. I was like, *OMG. This isn't happening.* So he hurried up, turned it off, and said, "Who turned that goofy channel on the television?"

Yes, up until this point, I thought my dad never looked at another woman besides my mom. I still like to think that. I think the porn channel episode was just a hotel glitch in the system. Goofy Arizona motels anyways. Too much sun out there is the problem. All that heat makes people crazy out there or something. Makes television electrical wires cross, too.

Washing my own towels was for the birds. I could never get them to come out of the wash as soft, as fluffy, and as fresh smelling as Mom could, so I flew home a week after Dad left. He needed some time off work anyway. Every guy needs some time away from work, away from cutting grass, to watch porn (just kidding, Dad).

My sister was furious. Furious isn't the word. She was totally pissed off at me. Finally, after eighteen F-in years of sharing a room with me, she gets her own room. She spent all week as happy as can be, organizing "her" room the way "she" wanted it. She had closet space now. She had room to put her things. Her teddy bear, Teddy, had his own chair with space to put his clothes. Teddy was happy. She was happy. Not anymore. She had to move everything. I think we didn't speak for a year. She was mad.

Especially the time I came home after a few too many beers, turned on the big overhead light while she was sleeping, and sat down at the makeup mirror and made myself into a unicorn with the hair mousse. I think even Teddy gave me a dirty look that night. Actually, Teddy's mouth was starting to peel off from wear and tear, but my sister wouldn't admit it. One Christmas, I made Teddy all these new mouths, but Lisa thought it was a dumb idea and threw them away. She holds grudges for long periods of time. Teddy doesn't, though. I know Teddy likes me.

My mom bought Teddy a tuxedo jacket to wear on the day of my wedding. We had a country western wedding.

Bill was the apple of my eye back in high school. There's no one in school who could write "Buck Naked" on the cheerleaders' signs in the hallway like Bill could. Bill taught me everything I know that's worth knowing. He taught me how to drink beer, go parking, and put a worm on a fishing hook. You know how to do those three things in life, you're going to lead one happy, fulfilled life. You see, life doesn't get any better than having a few beers, baiting your own hook, and parking your car in a secluded spot. Miss out on one of those and you'll end up on an antidepressant.

Everyone was excited about the country wedding. "Finally, a wedding we can wear jeans and cowboy boots to," many guests said.

Everyone except my mother-in-law. Bill's mom is extremely old-fashioned. You do everything the way everyone else does or else people will talk about you and you don't want people to talk about you. The first time I met my future mother-in-law, she came out of the bathroom without a shirt on. I thought I was going to die. I've never seen my own mom's boobs. She acted like it was nothing and walked across the room to get her shirt. I think my wedding plans gave her irritable bowel syndrome, among a few others things.

Chapter 11

We all need our doctors at some point or another. Some need their doctors more frequently than others. There are many wonderful doctors out there, taking care of us, also. Doctors mean well and do the best of what they can do to keep us healthy. And prescribing drugs to treat our symptoms is what they have all learned in medical school. However, we do need to keep in mind that doctors are in business. They are in business to not only take care of their patients but also to make money. If there was no financial incentive in any form of money or golf trips, vacations, lunches, dinners, etc., maybe your doctor would not prescribe a drug so readily. The idea to not offer financial incentives may help the American public, but it may also hurt the American public because it could deter the further development of medicine. For without the incentive of selling a new drug, the pharmaceutical companies may not invest in manufacturing new drugs to put on the market.

We have to note here, even with all the backlashing of prescription drugs, they are valuable aspects of our health and needed by many people. Dr. Marcia Angell, author of *The Truth About the Drug Companies: How They Deceive Us and What to Do About It*, is an outspoken proponent of medical and pharmaceutical reform. She was named one of the twenty-five most influential people in America by *Time* magazine. Although Dr. Angell proposes reform, she still recognizes the importance of medicine:

> This is not to gainsay the vital role of good prescription drugs in health care. There is no doubt that many people live longer, better lives because of them. . . But they should be prescribed carefully and only when necessary, and doctors' judgment about their prescription should be based on real research and education, not on the marketing that passes for it (172).

As important as medication can be, we do have to recognize that, usually, a pill (usually maintenance medication) treats the symptoms of an underlying problem. In essence, we are settling for living with our problem and taking a pill to alleviate some of the symptoms, or in the case of preventative medicine, we are taking a pill to prevent a more serious ailment that may occur. So, we are going to see a doctor or a specialist in hopes of getting rid of our problem, but instead, we are leaving the doctor's or specialist's office with the same problem we went in with, but with another pill to take. As discussed previously, this is what is taught at our medical schools. Our future doctors are taught a primarily science-based curriculum.

What if the curriculum of our medical schools was changed to reflect a more "healing-based" learning? If, let's just say, chiropractic medicine was combined with science-based medicine, then maybe less pain medication would be prescribed because a slight adjustment of the spine may be just what the doctor ordered. Or perhaps supplements and herbal medicine could be tried on a patient before a medication was prescribed for acid reflux. Acupuncture could be tried for many patients for various reasons, instead of a medicine cabinet full of pill bottles. The solution, ultimately, could be as simple as taking care of your own health by eating healthier and exercising.

From a business money-making point of view, this is not feasible because of all the lost profit of drug companies. We are looking at a 250-billion-dollar-revenue-generating industry (Carroll, 152). If you take the many small businesses of chiropractors, acupuncturists, naturalistic doctors, homeopathic doctors, etc. and had them donate to one central fund to try to get a bill passed in Congress to add their services as part of covered health care services, it probably wouldn't come close to the money that pharmaceutical companies would put forth to stop that from happening. Drug companies give generously to campaigns all the time. Drug companies gave approximately $85 million in the 1999-2000 elections (Angell, 200). And, "According to the consumer advocacy group Public Citizen, from 1997 through 2002, the industry spent nearly $478 million on lobbying" (Angell, 198).

Pharmaceutical companies spend a lot of money trying to get bills passed in their favor.

If drug companies do not foresee a profitable exchange for their drug endeavors, they would not continue to invest money in their efforts. Looking forward to current developments in the health care world in the book, *Reforming America's Health Care System: the Flawed Vision of Obamacare*, Scott Gottlieb, a resident fellow of the American Enterprise Institute, shows us how market outlook may affect the decisions to continue innovative drug programs:

> . . . drug companies are more frequently concluding that the additional cost of continuing development of a drug is not worth its projected returns. In turn, they are voluntarily canceling late stage programs. One older survey of this phenomenon found that between 1981 and 1992, more than 30 percent of curtailed drug programs were shuttered because of "economic reasons." The practice has only grown since (57).

It is clear that money is a major factor in the dispensing of prescription drugs. What drugs you need and take affect your health and your monthly budget. It is important to look out for yourself and your own well-being, keeping in mind that medicine is a business and is not always looking out for the best interest of your health.

It seems that one of the health problems of recent decades has been what has been referred to as acid reflux or heartburn. This problem seemed to have increased lately, possibly due to our dieting habits. Maybe we have made drive-thru dining a regular habit, but for whatever reason, Americans have been experiencing this ailment quite frequently. Nexium is a very popular expensive prescription drug used to treat this GERD disorder. The cause of GERD is not corrected by taking this medication, but rather, it helps in "suppressing stomach acid" (Critser, 198). For a lot of people who experience acid reflux symptoms or heartburn-like symptoms, taking Nexium or a similar pill provides much-needed relief. There are approximately 2.5 million Americans taking these GERD drugs daily (Critser, 198). So the question to ask is, is it beneficial to suppress stomach acid? Dr. Jonathan V. Wright, a clinician at the Tahoma Clinic in Kent, Washington, believes that a person with not enough stomach acid can develop problems with the digestion of essential minerals (Critser, 198-199). Dr. Wright's research showed that the patients who were taking GERD medications were in danger of eye degeneration and heart disease. Dr. Wright told his patients to stop taking the GERD medicine and, instead, take mineral supplements and hydrochloric acid. In doing this, Dr. Wright wanted to actually raise their stomach acid levels. "In almost all cases, the patients' problems resolved themselves" (Critser, 199).

This kind of research and use of alternative methods of health care could benefit many Americans and is a prime example of how people need to look out for their own health and not always accept what the doctor says. It may be that the doctor only knows one way to treat acid reflux or heartburn, and that is with a pill. Or his decision could be financially driven. Or it may even be that it's the quickest way to get you out of his office and on to the next patient. Americans tend to run to the doctors much more frequently than perhaps fifty years ago when a lot of the population was self-pay instead of insurance-pay. If we could eliminate just one pill from our ever-growing pillboxes, just think of the money we could save over a lifetime.

Chapter 12

After marriage and two kids, my days were long and busy. I spent the time reading to the kids, playing with them on the swing set, making sandwiches for Bill, doing laundry, and taking the kids to story time at the library. Nammy (Dalton's name for my mom) got off work at four o'clock. By now, Mom gave up on telemarketing and got a job as a secretary down the block. She walked to work every day, and at four o'clock, I would put Dalton in the stroller, we would walk down the block to Nam's work, and walk home with her. I think Dalton's first words were, "Is it four o'clock yet?"

My mom hated her job. I think it gave her a stomach ulcer.

One time, Mom and Dad were walking through the parking lot at Eat-N-Park and Mom just fell. Thank God Dad caught her. She just passed out. She didn't trip or anything. We went to visit her in the hospital and was like, "Mom, why did you pass out?"

She acted like it was nothing.

She just couldn't take out anytime for herself and go to the doctor because she was always too busy taking care of us. So every day, she'd get more lightheaded until finally, boom, she went down in the parking lot of Eat-N-Park.

Thank heavens my dad is so attuned to my mom. He's the true ladies' man, but only to one lady and one lady only, and that's my mom. I've never seen anything like it. He's like the perfect gentleman, like back in the old days, when opening the doors for the women was the most natural thing to do. He is always right there beside her, holding her hand, asking what he could do for her next, what she wants, and what he can get for her.

And dancing, dancing with my mom is his thing. He has dreams of being on *Dancing with the Stars* and the star is my mom. My dad got rhythm, too. He can dance like the black boys. It hasn't always been a stroll in the park, though, this whole dancing experiment. My dad expects to be perfect and my mom doesn't have every step down pat all the time, especially after she has a few drinks. My mom likes her rum and Cokes. That's just the way we roll.

After we moved out, Mom and Dad decided it's time to party, I guess. They have happy hour almost daily, they meet their friends at Legions, and they're out hitting the dance floor every weekend. My mom got all kinds of new clothes now. Dancing clothes, lower cut blouses, nice slacks, and ooh-so-fancy dancing shoes. Real dancing heels like the stars wear. There is some kind of cloth on the bottom so she can glide across the dance floor with my dad's rough, calloused hands holding her long, freckled, wrinkled fingers with her pink-painted long, thin, perfect nails.

They are one fine-looking couple. My mom and dad.

Thank goodness I found myself a nice man like my dad, because if I didn't, I may have had to sleep on the floor some nights. A few months after my daughter was born, my feet swelled. There were days I couldn't walk because the swelling was so great and it was very painful. So, I would crawl across the floor with Dalton and Lena. And when we needed something to eat or drink, I would pull myself up on my walker. It was tough getting to the grocery store and running errands. I had to wear big, arthritic tennis shoes, carry a baby, hold a walker, and keep track of my son running off. By the end of the day, I couldn't walk another step. Bill would come home from working second shift and find me lying somewhere in the house. Sometimes, I would be in the hallway. Sometimes, I would be at the top of the steps. It became a guessing game: "Where will Renee be lying tonight?"

Bill would scoop me up and carry me to bed. I took a lot of pills for my swollen feet: pain pills and steroids. The doctors couldn't figure out what was wrong. One day, Bill got tired of his wife not feeling well, and he called the doctor and told the doctor that he's taking me to the hospital so someone could figure out how to make me better. I remember lying in the hospital bed with my hospital robe on, no makeup on, my hair a mess, with five men staring at my feet and unshaven legs. How humiliating. Bill stood by our preacher. I don't know, but if the preacher is at your hospital bed, then something must not be good. But as I later found out, he was just passing through and happened to notice my name on the hospital list. Finally, after many tests, one of the doctors declared I had arthritis. Bill took me back home, and I continued to crawl across the floor and collapse somewhere at night. After seeing an acupuncturist, the pain and swelling went away.

When my son was young, he and my mom played with his little dirt bike motorcycles every day. One day, Nammy would pretend to be Travis Pastrana and Dalton would pretend to be Ricky Carmichael, and the next day, Nam would pretend to be Ricky Carmichael and Dalton would pretend to be Travis Pastrana. Nnnn, Nnnn, Nnnn. Crash.

"Are you all right, Travis?" Dalton would ask my mom.

Nnnn, Nnnn, Nnnn. Crash. "Are you all right, Ricky?" my mom would ask Dalton.

This is what they did. Almost every day. For years. Until one day, Dalton grew up. He started riding his own dirt bike. Nam didn't want to ride dirt bikes.

Nam didn't want to make my dad sandwiches, either.

Dad retired and didn't want to start another car project, either. So Dad went back to work and Mom said, "You're packing your own lunches."

Dad doesn't mind, though. As long as he still has my mom, he doesn't care that he has to make his own sandwiches.

Nam spends time with my daughter, Lena, now. They do crossword puzzles and talk about when they're going to clean Lena's closet. Then, after they finally clean Lena's closet, they talk about how her closet is going to stay organized for a long time. But a few weeks later, I go down to the swing and listen to Lena and Mom talk about when they are going to clean Lena's closet again.

Mom takes care of the kids for me when they're sick and have to stay home from school. Who else better to do the job than the expert? There's no comparing. She's the best. If you're sick, you're going to Nam's. Dalton and Lena know this.

Mom reads now. My dad leaves for work. And Mom reads. She reads all day. I don't even know if she stops to eat. She just reads. If I call her or if I stop by, she's reading. That's why I wrote this book: because I'm afraid she's running out of things to read, LOL. She reads novels, big novels, and has them done in two days. A day and a half sometimes. She ships books to California for her sister, Betty, to read. Betty probably has books stacked underneath her pool table, where the Dallas Cowboy Cheerleaders used to live. There's probably so many books that the pool table doesn't rest on its legs anymore. It's probably held up by books. As a matter of fact, I bet you can't even see the pool table anymore because there's so many books stacked around it. Mom takes boxes of books to Hoppy, her cigarette-smoking friend, from down the road. They probably smell like cigarettes when she gives them back. Mom takes books to her sister, Dorothy, who lives two streets down. And she sometimes gets in her car and drives to her other sister's house, about five miles away, and drops off boxes of books.

Mom also gives books to me and my sister, but only the ones she gives a "ten" to. Every book she reads, she writes her name in the inside cover and rates them one to ten. Lisa and I have enough books to take us well into retirement.

Maybe that's why Dad went back to work: to buy Mom books. I can see him now at the interview: "Paul, why do you want to return to work?"

My dad would clear his throat, put his leg up on his other leg, look up over his glasses, smile, and say, "My wife wants to read."

I don't know. Maybe my dad went back to work to pay for their prescriptions they have both accumulated through the years of raising my sister and me.

Chapter 13

Many Americans are taking too many prescription drugs because doctors, pharmaceutical companies, and pharmaceutical sales representatives are profiting. We need to lower the cost of prescription drugs for people who need them. Also, we need to educate consumers and doctors about alternative medicine so they can be aware of natural approaches to treat some health problems. The truth is our bodies and our wallets are affected by these drugs. We are told by our doctors that there is a pill for every problem. Our lives have become so fast-paced that we don't have time to contemplate our own health or the health of our family. Perhaps in the near future, we will have a drive-thru doctor's office where we can pull up to the window, press a button for what problem we are having, and, at the next window, a month's worth of pills will be distributed to us. And, unaware of what all of this medicine is doing to our bodies, we will swallow the pills.

Theoretically, let's suppose we are on prescription drugs that our bodies truly need. We, as Americans, budget our money to pay for all of our prescriptions and pay more for them than any other country. Most of us accumulate a new prescription every so many years.

However, when we retire and our income drops, we are supposed to continue to pay for all of our medications.

By taking control of our own health, we can limit the prescriptions we take; therefore, limiting the amount we pay out of our own pockets each year for our drugs. Something needs to be changed in order to alter the current dependency on prescription drugs. If a doctor weren't profiting by writing a prescription, he or she may or may not write that prescription for you. If drug companies weren't making a huge profit on a drug you heard about while you were watching your favorite television show, why would they spend thousands of dollars on advertising that particular drug?

In addition, if doctors were taught differently in medical school about finding a way to treat the actual disease instead of just treating the symptoms of the disease, this may limit the prescriptions we have to take throughout our lives. Exploring other options, such as supplements, herbs, chiropractic, or acupuncture may benefit some of us and, ultimately, reduce our need for some of our prescription drugs.

All of the above ideas need to be explored more closely in order to see if we can help our own health and the health of our nation as a whole, given the current state of our health care system and the future of our health care system. It is important that we all understand what is going on with our own bodies, as we have to be our own advocate.

We all have things from childhood we remember, and whether you're a mom, a dad, a grandpa, a grandma, an aunt, an uncle, a child, etc., you have these memories. These memories may make you laugh or they may make you cry. But every one of us has his or her own story: his or her own brick in the wall.

With all the iPods, iPhones, iPads, and iThings out there, we should take the time and listen to each other's stories. Behind every pill, there is a story.

Take, for instance, Willis from West Virginia. Willis lives in a very long ranch house which has a deck that extends the whole length of the house. There's a gate that wraps around Willis's two hundred acres so the sheep and cows don't get out. Willis lives so high up on a mountain in West Virginia that when it snows, the snowflakes are as big as your hand and they are also perfectly symmetrically shaped. The large snowflakes fall on the cows in the winter. The large snowflakes fall on the sheep in the winter. However, the large snowflakes do not fall on his pet pigs in the winter. Why? Well, because Willis's two pet pigs, Molly and Dolly, are in the house with him. Molly and Dolly take up a lot of space, too. Each weighs between three hundred to four hundred pounds. He feeds the pigs with cat food. Molly and Dolly eat a lot of cat food. Willis also has cows, but they are outside. One of the cows comes right up to the living room window and watches the news. Every day, the big jersey cow looks in Willis's window and watches the news with him. One day, Willis had some health issues and had to get a scooter to get around the house in. He was taking quite a few medications and couldn't really afford cat food anymore, so Willis had to make bacon. There may be no more Molly and Dolly, but there are still big snowflakes that fall on that West Virginia mountain.

Maybe you live in West Virginia next door to Willis. But you may not have known he had pet pigs.

You see your neighbor on occasion cutting their grass, getting in and out of their cars, but do you really know them? Sure, you may know where they work, but do you know anything about where they grew up, what their parents were like? The more you write or talk, the more interesting someone becomes.

For example, let's say you live next to Mr. Finkle. Mr. Finkle is always pulling in and out of his driveway every day, several times a day. You may wonder, where is Mr. Finkle going now? He just got home a few minutes ago. Maybe you didn't know that Mr. Finkle's wife is quite sick and he needs to pick up her prescriptions quite often. Or maybe you did know Mrs. Finkle is sick, but how many prescriptions can one person take? Where else can Mr. Finkle be going day after day? Well, what a lot of his neighbors don't know is that he won second place in his state's horseshoe-throwing tournament. Or when Mr. Finkle is not throwing horseshoes, he is oftentimes shooting squirrels. Mr. Finkle makes a fantastic dish called "microwaved squirrel meat with tomato sauce." Well, I'm actually going to just take his word that it is fantastic without actually trying it.

Sometimes, it takes all we have to afford our prescriptions. Some people need some help, because behind every expensive pill, there is a high co-pay. Take, for instance, Elva. Elva has a son, Brian, who is mentally handicapped. Elva plays the piano at her local church. Although her son was mentally challenged, he took care of his mother and she took care of him also. Every day, they had a routine that they would strictly adhere to. Finances got a little rough at times, and when Elva and her son needed a new roof, a giving neighbor paid for their roof to be shingled.

I'm not saying you have to be buy your neighbor a new roof, but that there may be help out there somewhere.

Do we all reach a point in our lives when we just get tired of paying for our prescriptions and we become "Ralph" and not say anything anymore? We stop complaining and become robots and just pay a higher price than the rest of the world for them? After all, bricks are quite silent. Even when rain hits them, there is no noise.

As Americans, are we settling for less than we should? Is there a point we reach where we have to stop "feeling comfortable"? This is not something we should get instantly angry about. After all, we've been "accepting" these costs for a long period of time now. It has been a gradual change. A dollar here and a dollar there. Then it became five dollars here and five dollars there. Then it became ten dollars here and ten dollars there. Then it became twenty dollars here and twenty dollars there. Actually, a lot of people pay around a forty-dollar co-pay for a one month's supply for a brand-name prescription. Some people on higher-priced drugs pay more. Or perhaps even full price for a drug if you do not have any prescription coverage. This could get very costly especially if your particular prescription costs hundreds of dollars.

It would probably not be a good idea to drive to the pharmacy, walk up to the pharmacist, and start yelling at him or her about how expensive your medication is. Nor would it be a good idea to keep a machete in your recliner chair like Ed from Jeannette.

Ed lives in a rather challenging neighborhood with drug dealers and women who sell themselves for drugs on the street corners. Ed lives in the first floor apartment with his pet cat, Snickers. Ed's apartment is one big room except for the bathroom. Ed's bed is in the back of the room and his living room is in the front of the room. There is no kitchen. Snickers is like Ed's best friend. He talks to Snickers all day. Every day. Ed seems so proud that he bought Snickers, his best buddy, a toy that he claims Snickers just loves and plays with. It is a blue circular tube that encloses a ball. Snicker chases the ball around the tube when she is not sitting at the windowsill, watching nonprescription and, possibly, prescription drugs exchange hands. Ed's wife passed away years ago, and his daughter met a man and moved to Arizona. Ed hopes he can save enough money to go to Arizona to visit his daughter. Ed doesn't like the tenants who live above him. He said they are drug dealers. Therefore, Ed keeps a machete in his living room recliner to protect himself and Snickers. Ed talks about packing his belongings to drive to Arizona with Snickers, of course. But, first, he has to save enough money to buy an old truck.

Looking at the world as a whole, not just America, do we really know who it is to blame for the high cost of prescription drugs? Think about it for a minute. We just automatically want to blame the big drug companies because we look at how much money they have and how much money they have made in the past year. After all, they do supply us with all the drugs that we need to stay alive, to function, or to get through life. So, perhaps we should not call them our enemy.

Let's say you get fired from work. You are going to want to know why. What it is that you did wrong. You are not going to want your boss to walk in and fire you for doing nothing wrong.

What needs to be done is to sit down and explain why costs are so high. If we don't play favorites, then something can be accomplished. It's hard for an elected official not to play favorites because of political contributions.

There are so many people involved in the costs of drugs that it may be a difficult task to actually place blame on any one entity. There are chemists, lab technicians, CEOs, doctors, pharmacists, researchers, etc. Now, after a price of a drug is decided upon, there are factors in deciding who is actually going to pay that exact price for that particular drug, and there are too many factors to even list. A person may qualify for a lower price because of a lower income. Or a person may not have drug coverage at all so the pharmaceutical company that manufactured the drug may help with the cost. There is a lot of subsidizing going on here, whether it be on the federal, state, or private level. In conclusion, some drug pricing is high and we are all suffering the consequences of high drug prices.

Life isn't fair, so no use getting ourselves all worked up about it (if we do, we might end up on another medication). It's a possibility that if there weren't constant battling over who is right and who is wrong, we may come to a logical solution to our problem.

We can all help one another. You can help your children or your grandchildren or your parents or your neighbor (and you don't even have to shingle your neighbor's roof). With lower drug costs, your neighbor might be able to afford to shingle his or her own roof.

Chapter 14

L ong before Walmart, in a little coal-mining town lived Grandma Lena and Grandpa. Company houses lined the seven streets of this little coal-mining town, where the men worked in the coal mine and the women tended to their families, husbands, and children. The owners of the coal mine not only owned the coal mine but also owned all of the houses, which looked identical to one another, and the company store. There was also a local tavern in town where all the men drank, shot pool, and played cards (for money). A lot went on in the little coal-mining town where everybody knew everyone. And when one of the men would have a little too much to drink, he would walk up and down the streets trying to find his home. It was not unusual for one of the men to walk into another family's home, thinking it was his own. Also, it was not unusual for one of the women to chase the lost man out of her home with a pan or a rolling pin if her husband was not home.

Grandpa was a very good pool shooter and oftentimes tried to bet some of his paycheck from the mine on a game of pool. Grandma Lena, like all of the other miners' wives, knew when it was payday. The owners of the coal company also acted as "the bank," so the miners didn't have to go home to cash their paychecks. They would head straight to the tavern. There were many times when Grandma Lena sent my dad down the road to the tavern to fetch my grandpa before all of his money was gone. My dad's knees would shake as he walked down the road, scared to death of telling my grandpa that it was time to leave the tavern and come home now.

With the money that was left, the rent had to be paid to the coal mining company and food had to be bought from the company store. Grandma Lena had to pack "dinner buckets," which was what they used to call lunches, for Grandpa and his two younger brothers, who also worked in the mine but didn't have wives to tell them that it was time to come home before they gambled their paychecks away. Every day, Grandpa's brothers took their dinner buckets to work until one day, my grandpa found out through the grapevine (it's a small world after all) that his brothers were selling their dinner buckets for money to spend at the tavern. That was the end of Grandma Lena's subsidization.

In the New Testament, an "early church" was established in a small community. Everyone pulled their resources together and distributed them to all members as needed. There was a "common pot" and all had enough to care for themselves. This could be likened to what is now "subsidizing" drug costs. But the issue here is, does the idea of "subsidizing" work for everybody?

Let's take, for example, a lady named Rose. Rose's husband worked very hard all his life. He raised a family the best he could even though Rose's husband didn't make it to all of the kids' ballgames because of his long working hours. The kids grew up and Rose's husband had a heart attack and passed away. Rose went to work long hours to make up for the loss of income. Now, Rose is getting older. She's now paying higher costs for her health care and her medications: something she is not used to doing when her husband was alive and carried work benefits. In addition, her health is not as good as it was when she was younger. So, she's now visiting the doctors more frequently, and being prescribed more drugs, which results in more out-of-pocket costs for Rose.

Now, back to the "Early Church." If you were Rose, what do you feel would be the fair thing to do?

1. Lower Rose's prescription costs by more subsidization,
2. Keep the "status quo," or
3. Make Rose pay more for her prescriptions.

The "Early Church" scenario protects against some becoming incredibly rich or incredibly poor. It sounds like a fair concept. For a while anyway. Until time goes on. Time passes. You work. You work harder. And you work even harder. And then you may say, "Wait a minute. Something is not fair here." Rose and her husband worked hard their whole lives. By more subsidization, maybe Rose's drugs will be less; however, that money is going to have to come from somewhere. So maybe Rose will have to pay more taxes, so there is more in the "common pot." It's almost like your robbing Peter to pay Paul. The consensus among many of the baby boomers I have spoken to is this: they have saved what they "thought" would be enough for retirement; however, what they didn't factor in was the additional monies that would go to prescription drug costs. During the ten-year period from 1999 to 2009, there was a 39% increase in the number of prescriptions dispensed (population growth was 9%) (Lundy, 3).

Going back to our "Behind every pill, there is a story" philosophy, the bottom line here is now that Rose is on more prescriptions than she was a few years ago and her out-of-pocket costs are higher now than in years past, she now has less money left over every month to pay for flowers for her flower garden. And what makes Rose happy? A pretty yard.

Chapter 15

My grandpa always told me, "Never get old, Nay. Never get old."

Whenever my Uncle Fred, Aunt Aileen, and Cousin John visited, John, Lisa, and I pretended to be spies. John would tell Lisa she was to hide behind Grandpa's kitchen sink, I was to hide under Grandpa's kitchen table, and he was to hide behind Grandpa's kitchen cabinet. We would all run across the tiny hallway over to Grandpa's side of the house and take our appropriate spots. Then, we would all take turns sneaking up to the living room door where Grandpa, my dad, and Uncle Fred were talking. Talking about politics, of course. Each would yell at the other over this problem and that problem. It all seemed so interesting. They would take turns yelling back and forth at each other.

We wanted to hear what it was they were yelling about. The game was all so suspenseful. We didn't want to get caught. We pretended that we were government spies on a mission. My heart would beat faster and faster when it was my turn to peak in the door and find out what they were saying. I would slowly try to get out from under the green-painted wooden table and chairs without making a noise. Lisa and John would be looking at me with smiles on their faces, trying so hard not to laugh. If I accidentally bumped the table or chairs, they would cover their mouth with their hands so they could stop themselves from laughing. On the tips of my toes, I would creep over to the door with my number two pencil and tablet paper in my hand. Then, I would write down things I heard my grandpa, dad, and Uncle Fred say, "It's those Democrats . . ." my grandpa would say.

"It's the Republicans . . ." my dad would say.

After we all took our turns at spying, the three of us would run as fast as we could through the little hallway, which separated the duplex, back to the kitchen on our side of the house. Out of breath, we would roll around, laughing hysterically at our accomplishments. Then, we would recount to each other everything we thought we heard from the living room and how Lisa almost got caught because she bumped the side of the cabinet with her foot. The adult conversation was always about current world affairs and their opinions on which elected official was making the right and wrong decisions.

As a matter of fact, each election day, my grandpa would put his fancy hat on and down the road he would walk to vote. He was so proud to vote. It was a very important day: Election Day. Not something that you attempt to fit in your schedule. When it was an election day, that was the first and foremost important thing to do that particular day. So after the soggy cornflakes and egg were eaten, and after the insulin shot was given, down the road went Grandpa, with his fancy hat on, to vote.

Walking down the road a few blocks to vote must have taken a lot out of Grandpa because he would sleep most of the afternoon after voting. In good weather, Grandpa slept sitting up in his chair outside, facing the road, with Kitty on the porch above him sleeping, too. The two of them did a lot of napping. People drove up and down the road and beeped their horns at Grandpa. He would awaken startled and wave to the passing vehicles. Then he would ask me, "Hey, Nay, who was that?"

And I would always say, "I don't know, Grandpa."

I never really knew anybody who waved to Grandpa in the passing cars, but it never failed; Grandpa would still ask me, "Hey, Nay, who was that?"

In the winter months, Grandpa also enjoyed napping a lot. He had a chair that was beside his living room window. He watched television and then stared out the window until he fell asleep. When Kitty was outside, she would hop up to the windowsill and fall asleep with Grandpa. When I was outside and Grandpa and Kitty were sleeping, I would tap on the window, and the tapping noise would startle him. He would smile and wave his hand just like he did to the passing cars. Except he knew who I was.

There were days when I was older when my mom and dad would leave me home alone. I would walk through the little hallway that separated our side of the house and Grandpa's, and sit on a chair in his living room and watch television with him. He was always watching animal shows. Shows about wildlife. Survival of animals in the wild. I remember most of the animals lived in a pack. They took care of their children and each other. The males guarded the group against other packs and predators. They looked after one another and made sure each had enough to eat. Grandpa and I would eventually fall asleep.

Grandpa was sleeping the morning I was leaving for Arizona for college. It was very early in the morning and I slowly opened the painted white wooden door that led to the painted brown wooden, creaky steps. I slowly walked up the steps on the tips of my toes to Grandpa's bedroom. He was sleeping. I gave him a kiss on his cheek and rubbed the palm of my hand on the top of his head. I did this all the time when I was a kid. Grandpa used to come home from the barber shop with a crew cut (the kind you get in the military). He would bend down and I would graze the palm of my hand over his crew cut and laugh. It felt so funny. It tickled my hand. I would laugh. Grandpa would laugh.

Grandpa awoke when I did this the morning I left for Arizona for college and said, "Hey, Nay, why do you have to go so far away to college?"

"I don't know," I told Grandpa.

"I love you, Nay," he said.

I turned away and tip-toed back down the creaky, brown-painted wooden steps, shut the painted white wooden door, and unknowingly latched the door lock.

Poor Grandpa was locked upstairs all day without his soggy cornflakes, egg, and insulin shot until the rest of the family got home from the airport. Oops, sorry, Grandpa.

Grandpa was in and out of the hospital a lot over the next two years. He didn't awaken when I tapped on the windowsill anymore. In the summers, he didn't awaken when people drove by and beeped their horns at him, either.

One day, I came home from the local mall where I was working at a bakeshop and I said, "Where's Grandpa?"

My dad said that he and Uncle Fred had to take Grandpa to a nursing home. So every day after all of the bread, buns, and sweet rolls were baked, I left the bakeshop to visit Grandpa at the nursing home.

Grandpa seemed to not get much attention at the nursing home. He would just lie there in bed. When I was at the nursing home visiting, a nurse would deliver his food and pills to him on a tray, and the tray would just sit there untouched. I would say, "Grandpa, aren't you hungry?" Or, "Grandpa, do you want to take your pills?"

He would say, "No."

Each day after baking at the mall, I would go to the nursing home to sit with Grandpa, and each day, he would not eat or take his pills. I would hold his cup of cold coffee for him to drink with a straw. His dry, chapped lips could hardly fit around the straw to drink. It took a long time to drink one cup of coffee, but I didn't mind, as long as Grandpa was happy with his coffee. Sometimes, after drinking the coffee, we would both fall asleep together.

One day, though, I got mad. I got mad at the nurses who were not taking care of my grandpa. This is my grandfather. The man who made me laugh with his crew cuts. The man with shiny black shoes who danced to "Rag Time Cowboy Joe." The man who voted every

Election Day. The man who went to honor our veterans at all of the Memorial Day and Veterans Day celebrations. Doesn't my grandpa deserve better care than this? I left Grandpa's hospital bed, walked down the hall to find the nurse, and said to the nurse, "My grandpa hasn't eaten or taken his pills for almost a week. If it weren't for me, he wouldn't have anything to drink, either."

She stopped, looked at me, and said, "I'm very sorry, but I'm the only nurse on this shift and I have twenty other patients to take care of."

And then she walked away.

My grandpa passed away that evening.

Sometimes, behind every pill, there is a sad story, too.

Works Cited

Altman, Stuart H. and David Shactman; foreword by John Kerry. *Power, Politics, and Universal Health Care: The Inside Story of a Century-Long Battle.* Amherst, N.Y.: Prometheus Books, 2011. Print.

Angell, Marcia. *The Truth About the Drug Companies: How They Deceive Us and What to Do About It.* New York: Random House, c2004. Print.

Atlas, Scott W., ed. *Reforming America's Health Care System: The Flawed Vision of Obamacare.* Stanford, Calif.: Hoover Institution Press, c2010. Print.

Barr, Donald A. "Revolution or Evolution? Putting the Flexner Report in Context." *Medical Education* 45.1 (2011): 17 – 22. *Academic Search Elite.* Web, 17 September 2012.

Carroll, Jamuna, ed. *The Pharmaceutical Industry.* Detroit: Greenhaven Press, c2009. Print.

Critser, Greg. *Generation Rx: How Prescription Drugs Are Altering American Lives, Minds, and Bodies.* Boston: Houghton Mifflin, 2005. Print.

DeNoon, Daniel. "The 10 Most Prescribed Drugs." *WebMD.* 2011: 1 – 2. Web, 3 July 2012.

Dietz, Elizabeth. *Trends in Employer-Provided*

Prescription-Drug Coverage. Monthly Labor Review Online. Bureau of Labor Statistics. Web, August 2004. Vol. 127, No. 8.

"Focus On Prices and Spending." *Consumer Expenditure Survey*, 2009. U.S. Bureau of Labor Statistics. Web, August 2011. Vol. 2, No. 8.

Gottfried, Dennis. *Too Much Medicine: A Doctor's Prescription for Better and More Affordable Health Care*. St. Paul, MN: Paragon House, 2009. Print.

Lundy, Janet. "Prescription Drug Trends." Kaiser Family Foundation. P3. N.d. Web, 24 June 2012.

Otfinoski, Steven. *Charles Drew*. New York: Macmillan/McGraw-Hill. P3. Print.

"Sacramento Man Indicted for Using Craigslist to Traffic in Counterfeit Viagra from China." FBI. U.S. Attorney's Office. Eastern District of California. Web, June 24, 2011.

Sager, Alan. "Affordable Medications for Americans." n.p. n.d. Web, 29 June 2012.

"Six Prescriptions for Change." *Consumer Reports*. 73.3 (2008): 14. *MasterFILE Premier*. Web, 17 September 2012.

"US Care Unwell Japan's Health Efficiency." *Herald Sun* (Australia). May 5, 2012. *LexisNexis*. Web, 17 September 2012.

Verbruggen, Damien B., ed. *Reforming America's Health Care System*. New York: Nova Science Publishers, Inc., c2010. Print.

www.ingramcontent.com/pod-product-compliance
Lightning Source LLC
Chambersburg PA
CBHW031948070426
42453CB00006BA/310